Chemotherapy Relief

(A short booklet – 8000+ words)

Chemotherapy research results
to protect you from chemo side effects

Chemotherapy Self-Help Series

Joyce Zborower, M.A.

ISBN-13: 978-1532909139
ISBN-10: 1532909136

Joyce Zborower, M.A.

For Chemo Turban Hats
And other Chemotherapy Patient Supplies
Visit

http://headgearexpress.com

Table of Contents

What Is Cancer

Cancer is a group of disease processes characterized by uncontrolled cell growth coupled with a tendency to become progressively worse (malignancy) with a proclivity to invade other areas of the body and develop secondary malignant growths some distance from the primary site of the disease (metastasis).

Cancer = uncontrolled cell growth + malignancy + metastasis

Cancer is the second leading cause of death in the United States. However, recent improvements in identifying its presence (detection), identifying its distinctive characteristics (diagnosis), and applying the necessary and appropriate treatment(s) have tended to increase survival rates for many people dealing with this disease.

To understand cancer, it is helpful to learn what happens to normal cells when they become cancerous. Normal growth is the result of normal cells growing and dividing and supporting normal body functioning. Sometimes something during this process causes the body to produce new cells when and where the body does not need them. At the same time, old cells in those areas do not die when they should. These extra cells form a cell mass and this cell mass is called a tumor. There are two types of tumors: benign tumors which do not include malignancy and metastasis (these are NOT cancer) and malignant tumors which divide without control or order, invade and destroy normal tissues around them, and can break away from their starting point and develop secondary malignant growths some distance away (these ARE cancerous).

Cancers are given different names and different treatments depending on where in the body they form. For example, malignant tumors forming in the breast are called breast cancer; malignant cancers forming in the groin or prostate area are called prostate cancers. Treatments for each type of cancer can differ.

Cancer treatment can include surgery, radiation therapy, chemotherapy, hormone therapy, and biological therapy – either alone or in combination with other treatments. Cancer treatments can damage healthy cells and tissues and often causes deleterious side effects. It is important for patients along with their doctors to weight the benefits of killing the cancerous cells against the risks of these possible side effects.

This booklet is not intended to be all-inclusive in discussing dealing with all the side effects produced by all of the various different cancer treatments. We will deal here with the deleterious side effects caused by chemotherapy and how to mitigate their effects.

References

Bellenir, Karen, Editor. *Cancer Sourcebook*, sixth edition. *Health Reference Series*. Peter E. Ruffner, Publisher. Copyright © 2011 by Omnigraphics, Inc.

http://en.wikipedia.org/wiki/Chemotherapy

What Is Chemotherapy

Chemotherapy (AKA chemo and/or CTX or CTx) is one of the treatments for cancer that uses chemical substances (drugs) to kill cancer cells. They interrupt the cancer cell's ability to replicate. These drugs tend to target cells that divide quickly, which means that healthy cells can also be harmed. Doctors can elect to use one drug or a combination of drugs to achieve the desired results. The desired result is not always that the cancer be cured though that could be what the doctor is looking to do. He/she may just be trying to prolong the patient's life by slowing the cancer's growth or to keep it from spreading or just to reduce the severity of symptoms.

The side effects of chemotherapy depend primarily on the type of drug(s) administered and the amount of that drug that is given. Chemotherapy side effects are caused by the chemo drugs harming healthy cells and can either be acute (short duration) or chronic (long duration).

Side effects can include:

Alopecia – Hair loss – a common side effect but not necessarily universal. Women are more likely to lose their hair than men. Use of a cold cap during chemo may help prevent alopecia of the scalp. More on this later.

Decreased production of blood cells – both red and white cells and platelets (myelosuppression). – may require specialized shots. Your doctor will talk with you if you need them.

Decreased immune system (immunosuppression) -- Your doctor should talk with you about this.

Typhlitis – a possible life threatening gastrointestinal complication brought on by chemotherapy. It is a medical emergency and often fatal unless dealt with quickly

Gastrointestinal distress – Inflammation of the lining of the digestive tract -- including "nausea, vomiting, anorexia, abdominal cramps and constipation." Antiemetic drugs (drugs that help to stop nausea and vomiting – typically drugs used to treat motion sickness) may help with these side effects. Also, patients may be told to eat frequent small meals and drink clear liquids and/or ginger tea. Do contact your doctor, however, as these are the same symptoms as typhlitis (above).

Anemia causing temporary fatigue – medical treatments to alleviate anemia include hormones to boost blood production, iron supplements, and blood transfusions. Your doctor should also check for thyroid problems in relation to fatigue. According to research, "women who get regular exercise during cancer treatment feel better and have more energy." Regular exercise can consist of walking 30 minutes per day, 3 – 4 days per week.

Poor appetite – Smoking medical marijuana is said to help alleviate cancer patients' poor appetite. At time of this writing, medical marijuana is legal in 23 states and the District of Columbia. It is pending in 3 others. You can get the latest information here:
http://medicalmarijuana.procon.org/view.resource.php?re sourceID=000881

Nausea and vomiting -- Drugs that prevent or reduce nausea or vomiting can usually help with those two side effects. "Some studies and patient groups say that the use of cannabinoids derived from cannabis during chemotherapy greatly reduces the associated nausea and vomiting, and enables the patient to eat." Use of ginger to control nausea and vomiting, though wide spread, is provided mixed support by the literature.

Diarrhea – consult with your doctor about this.

Secondary neoplasia – which is the formation or presence of a new, abnormal growth of tissue in a new place. Neoplasias can be either benign or malignant. People with childhood cancers are more likely to get secondary neoplasias.

Infertility – Some chemotherapy drugs are high risk for gonadotoxic effects while others are very low risk. Cryopreservation (freezing) of semen, eggs, oocytes (an ovarian cell capable of dividing) or embryos prior to chemotherapy is an option. Discuss this with your doctor prior to beginning chemotherapy treatments.

Sexual impotence – discuss this with your doctor.

Teratogenicity – which is the ability to cause malformation of a developing fetus (i.e., produces birth defects) especially in the first trimester in which case, abortions are usually recommended. Classes of teratogens include radiation, maternal infections, chemicals and drugs.

Peripheral neuropathy can be another side effect of chemotherapy. It consists of pain, numbness, tingling, and sensitivity to cold beginning in the extremities of hands and feet and can progress into the arms and legs. It is generally thought to be "progressive, enduring, and often irreversible." It is usually treated with drugs. However, a new, non-invasive treatment called KLaser is showing some promise here. More on this later.

Cognitive impairment – or reported inability to concentrate. Sometimes called "chemo brain". Some things to help alleviate chemo brain include:
 Exercise – this provides more oxygen to your brain
 Drink less alcohol
 Use fewer stimulants – caffeine and nicotine tend to produce anxiety which makes concentration difficult and may also interfere with sleep.
 Wear your glasses and hearing aid if needed.
 Minimize distractions

Tumor-lysis syndrome – is a potentially life threatening condition caused by the rapid break down of cancer cells releasing copious amounts of chemicals (uric acid, potassium, phosphate) into the blood stream.

Organ damage – Chemotherapy can produce heart damage, liver damage, kidney damage, nerve damage, and damage to reproductive organs as well as possible damage to the inner ear producing dizziness and/or vertigo.

Mouth and/or lip sores – a common problem with several kinds of chemotherapy. Recommendations for relief include "sucking on ice pops or ice chips and dabbing vitamin E oil on sore areas."

Red skin (erythema) – can also include peeling on the palms of your hands and/or the soles of your feet. It's a sunburn-like reaction to certain chemo drugs. Thick emollient creams can be spread on these areas several times per day. Wear loose socks or gloves to bed over the creams. Taking vitamin B_6 supplements may also help. If none of these help, your doctor may wish to change your dosage or give you more "time off" with this drug.

Dry skin – Chemo drugs seem to dry your skin and make it more sensitive. It may even cause rashes. Choose gentle non-perfumed products or those for sensitive skin. Use the products at the sales counter before purchasing to feel and see how they perform on your skin. Different people react to different products in different ways. Tell the salesperson you are undergoing cancer treatments. You can sparingly use serums designed to treat lower layer of skin prior to applying moisturizer. Exfoliations help remove dead skin cells. Creamy face masks help hydrate your skin and are good for dry skin. They can be used once or twice per week.
While doing chemo your skin may become sun sensitive – so wear at least a factor 15 sun block. Avoid swimming during chemo as dry skin tends to get dryer. Check with your doctor before using creams or lotions on areas undergoing radiation treatments.

Damaged fingernails – to reduce the possibility of nail damage during treatment, cold mittens can be placed on the hands and feet. More on this later.

Dry mouth – suck on ice chips. Sometimes sucking on hard candies is recommended but I think that's probably not a good idea as cancer has a "sweet tooth" and hard candies just might feed the cancer. Diabetes might also be an issue with hard candies. More on this later.

Water retention – AKA, lymphodemia. This side effect is thoroughly discussed in one of the sections that follow this general discussion.

Allergic or pseudo-allergic reactions – best to discuss these issues with your doctor.

Many of the above side effects can only be ameliorated with other medical interventions. We've provided only bare bones information regarding these. You should always speak with your doctor about all issues related to your chemotherapy treatments, however if you feel that those specific serious side effects are affecting you, call your doctor or speak with an appropriate health care provider immediately. Some of them can be lethal if not caught early.

We will be discussing other help for many of the less critical, but still annoying side effects later in this booklet.

Normal cells usually recover soon after chemotherapy ends so most chemotherapy side effects are not permanent and go away with the cessation of treatment. However, some side effects do not go away so easily. Some never go away.

It must also be noted that chemotherapy does not always provide the expected results.

So, to recap, the three benefits that can be derived from participating in the chemotherapy treatments are:
.....Curing your cancer
   Prolonging your life by slowing the growth of the cancer and keeping it from spreading
   Reducing the severity of the symptoms which includes reducing pain

Chemotherapy side effects are caused by the chemo drugs harming healthy cells and can either be acute or chronic.

There are at least 24 possible side effects to the procedure that must be considered in relation to the advantages/benefits when deciding whether or not to participate – some of which can be life threatening. This booklet does not and cannot deal specifically with the more serious complications of this procedure. If you believe any of these pertain to you and your situation, consult your doctor or health care professional.

This booklet provides suggestions for ways to improve your overall health – thus helping you cope with the overall procedure – as well as various things you can do to help your body deal with some of the less serious, but still annoying and deleterious, side effects of chemotherapy.

References

Bellenir, Karen, Editor. *Cancer Sourcebook*, sixth edition. *Health Reference Series*. Peter E. Ruffner, Publisher. Copyright © 2011 by Omnigraphics, Inc.

http://www.mayoclinic.org/tests-procedures/chemotherapy/basics/definition/PRC-20023578

http://en.wikipedia.org/wiki/Chemotherapy

Block, Keith I, M.D. *Life Over Cancer*: The Block Center Program for Integrative Cancer Treatment. Bantam Books. Copyright © 2009 by Keith I. Block, M.D.

McKay, Judith, RN, OCN. And Tamera Schacher, RN, OCN, MSN. *The Chemotherapy Survival Guide*, 3rd Edition. New harbinger Publication, Inc. Copyright © 2009 by Judith McKay and Tamera Schacher.

http://www.cancerresearchuk.org/about-cancer/cancers-in-general/treatment/cancer-drugs/side-effects/your-skin-nails-and-cancer-drugs

Clean Diet and Exercise

Two of the very best things you can do for yourself, whether you have cancer or not, is to
1. clean up your diet and
2. start walking at least 30 minutes per day 3 or 4 days per week. Using a walker is okay.

Cleaning up your diet means cutting down on or eliminating "junk food", chemical food additives, preservatives, processed foods, anything white that can go in your mouth like salt, sugar, and white flour. Start using natural sweeteners like honey, maple syrup, molasses, or date sugar. Substantially increase your Omega-3 intake with foods like flaxseed and walnuts as well as green leafy vegetables such as Brussels sprouts, kale, spinach, and salad greens. Some fish are also rich in Omega-3 fatty acids.

"Omega-3s can reverse tumor metastasis as well as a tumor's resistance to radiation or chemotherapy, and may also enhance chemo's effectiveness and minimize the toxic side effects of some chemotherapy drugs." Omega-3s are anti-inflammatory (reduces inflammation) and anti-thrombotic (reduces the possibility of blood clots). Omega-9 fatty acids (olive oil) are also beneficial. Omega-6s are essential for health but are less beneficial for cancer patients. They are proinflammatory (increases inflammation) and prothrombotic (an abnormality of blood coagulation which increases the possibility of blood clots).

According to Dr. Keith I. Block in his book *Life Over Cancer: The Block Center Program for Integrative Cancer Treatment*, says that "certain foods can inhibit cancer while others can encourage its survival and spread . . . and a thoroughly mundane activity like eating can be a powerful anti-cancer treatment. . . It boosts your energy so you have the stamina for radiation and chemo; it deprives the tumor of compounds it feeds on; it fills you with nutrients that keep malignant cells in check. And it epitomizes the integrative approach to cancer"

To the point that "what you eat can spell the difference between conquering your disease and having it rage out of control", Dr. Block developed his anti-cancer diet consisting of "low fat, high fiber . . . whole grains, fruits, vegetables, and legumes, plus foods rich in anti-cancer nutrients such as shitake mushrooms, sea vegetables, ginger, and green tea." The elimination of "all dairy, meat, and refined sugars" is also encouraged. However, diet alone is not to be regarded as the sole cancer fighting agent. "...(C)ombining conventional treatments with complimentary therapies in an integrative system buys the best odds for a successful outcome."

[For comprehensive food guidelines and sample meal plans for cancer patients, see chapter 5 (pp. 77 – 118) of Dr. Block's book, *Life Over Cancer*]

Exercise in the form of walking 30 minutes per day, 3 – 4 days per week "is correlated with a 50% decline in mortality in breast cancer patients. . . . Moreover, numerous studies show that inactivity can result in frailty, fatigue, and the loss of critical lean muscle; it can disrupt sleep cycles and impair tolerance and response to cancer treatment." Dr. Block goes on to emphasize that "exercise may be critical to your very survival."

It seems to me that if ***that*** doesn't get you moving, nothing will.

References

Block, Keith I, M.D. *Life Over Cancer:* The Block Center Program for Integrative Cancer Treatment. Bantam Books. Copyright © 2009 by Keith I. Block, M.D.

Start a Gratitude Journal

Your physical well-being is only part of the health and wellness picture. Mental health and mental attitude is a huge part of someone's feeling content and happy and good about one's self. And feeling good about one's self goes a long way towards feeling good about others and having a positive attitude about your specific circumstances. And having a positive attitude helps you be more giving and caring and – yes – likeable. People like to help people that they like.

Remember the old adage: you gather more flies with honey than with vinegar. Nobody likes to be around someone who's a "Debby Downer", i.e. someone who's negative and complaining all the time.

One of the best ways to keep a positive attitude – or improve a negative one – is to consciously record good things that happen to you during the day. Every day, not just once in a while. And a good way to remember and consciously record the day's good events – the things that you're grateful for and that make you feel good – is to keep a gratitude journal.

And it's easy. Writing about 5 good things that happened during the day that you're grateful for only takes about 5 or 10 minutes at night before you go to bed. And the things you're grateful for don't have to be big things. They can be, but they don't have to be. They can be something as simple as "I'm grateful I was able to get a full night's sleep last night." Or "I'm grateful the dog let me know when he had to go outside and didn't do his business in the house." Little good feelings add up to lots of positive feelings that make the rest of your life a little more enjoyable.

Your journal – the thing that you write in – can be as simple as a yellow pad of paper or as fancy as going to the store and buying a fancy notebook or diary especially to use as your gratitude journal. And after you've written several days worth of good feelings, you can re-read everything you've written and feel good all over again!

Alopecia -- Hair Loss

Hair loss seems to be a usual expectation of chemotherapy treatment but the newer single-agent chemotherapy drugs for advanced breast cancer don't necessarily produce this side effect. If that's the kind of treatment you're getting, you may not be troubled by any hair loss at all.

If you are getting treatments that do affect your hair, know that this hair loss is temporary and that your hair will begin growing back a few weeks after treatment ends though this may take several months and your new hair may be softer or curlier or a different color.

You might experience just thinning of hair or just losing hair patches or fairly total hair loss including scalp hair, eyebrows, eyelashes, and some to all of your body hair. There are a number of things you can do to help yourself feel better about it.

Speak with your doctor about something called a "cold cap". It's a special device that fits over your head while getting treatments that lowers the temperature of your scalp. This reduces the blood flow to the scalp thereby reducing the amount of drug that reaches the hair follicles. Though not guaranteed, this could help to make the hair less likely to die and fall out. However, there are some drawbacks to using a cold cap.

It makes you feel cold all over.

You have to spend longer at the hospital because it takes a while to cool your scalp before treatments can begin.

It could give you a headache.

It might not work and your hair could all fall out anyway.

For complete scalp hair loss:

If your hair is going to fall out, it usually begins 2 – 3 weeks after treatment starts. Loss tends to be gradual.

Wear a hairnet to bed so there isn't hair all over your pillow when you wake up.

You may wish to get a short haircut before treatment starts.

Some people choose to shave their heads to avoid seeing their hair fall out.

Wigs and scarves and hats and ball caps are obvious choices for hiding a bare head. If choosing a wig, you may wish to begin your search prior to beginning treatments. That way you can more easily match the color of the wig to the natural color of your hair.

This could be a good time to dramatically change your appearance by choosing a wig the color and style you've always wanted.

Some people choose to just go bald.

For partial scalp hair loss:

Depending on how much hair is lost and whether or not the remaining hair is still well-attached, some very gentle hair extensions might work to fill in lost patches or provide a thicker, fuller look to the hair that's left.

Be very gentle with the hair that's left.

Use a gentle baby shampoo and pat your hair dry instead of rubbing it.

Use a soft baby brush to brush your hair.

Avoid hair dryers and curling irons on thinning hair.

Avoid perms and hair color.

Using makeup to disguise the loss of eyebrows or eyelashes can help with feelings of acceptance. Buy products prior to starting treatment as treatments tend to tire you out and you may not feel like shopping after treatments begin. Buy colors close to your natural color. Practice using the makeup before losing your hair.

It is important to check with your doctor before using these products if:
　　You are still having cancer treatments.
　　Have had treatments to your face or neck.
　　Have had a skin reaction.

For loss of eyebrows:

Use an eye primer first to help makeup stay on longer.
Eyebrow stencil packs – include different size stencils, small brush, pencil, highlighters
Eyebrow kits – include wax and shadow
Eyebrow pencils – practice drawing eyebrows on your arm.

For loss of eyelashes:

Use an eye primer first to help makeup stay on longer.
Eyeliner pencil – choose a soft pencil as the skin around the eye is very sensitive.
Eye shadows – apply as eyeliner or to whole upper lid.
Gel eyeliner – lasts longer than pencil but is harder to put on.
False eyelashes – difficult to put on and keep on. Eyelash glue may irritate your skin. Especially hard to use if you've lost all your own lashes or have watery eyes. If you have any lashes left, removing false lashes might pull them out.

Many women going through chemotherapy treatments have found that full makeovers (hair, makeup, new clothes, etc.) can provide a real lift to their spirits and help them feel pretty and feminine again.

References

http://www.cancerresearchuk.org/about-cancer/cancers-in-general/treatment/cancer-drugs/side-effects/hair-loss-hair-thinning-and-cancer-drugs#wig

http://www.cancerresearchuk.org/about-cancer/coping-with-cancer/coping-physically/changes-to-your-appearance-due-to-cancer/tips-on-skin-care-and-make-up/eyelashes-how-to-define-your-eyes

Peripheral Neuropathy

Peripheral neuropathy is a chemo side effect manifested as nerve damage that can be brought on by or made worse by various chemotherapy drugs. Its symptoms include: pain, numbness, tingling, and sometimes sensitivity to cold. The symptoms generally begin in the extremities of hands and feet and can progress into the arms and legs. When caused by chemotherapy drugs, peripheral neuropathy is often temporary and tends to go away after a few weeks or months after stopping treatment but sometimes the residual effects last a lot longer.

Chronic peripheral neuropathy has no cure but there are remedies that can help. These remedies include: nutritional supplements (Vitamin B Complex mixture of all B vitamins, L-Glutamine and R-alpha-lipoic acid), medications (Neurontin, Elavil, Effexor, Tylenol, Motrin, Advil, hydrocodone, oxycodone), acupuncture, physical therapy, and gentle massage.

Food allergy studies have shown chronic peripheral neuropathy can be a manifestation of Celiac Disease.

If you are showing symptoms of peripheral neuropathy, here are a few things you should avoid:
   MSG (monosodium glutamate) – exacerbates neuropathy
   Wheat products -- gluten
   Simple sugars – white flour, white refined sugar, refined carbohydrates
   Statin drugs – cholesterol medications – exacerbates neuropathy
   Organic solvents – dry cleaning chemicals, glues, detergents, nail polish removers, etc.

Pesticides – eat these as organic products – apples, celery, strawberries, peaches, spinach, nectarines, grapes, sweet bell peppers, potatoes, blueberries, lettuce, Kale/collard greens
Coffee, soda pop, dairy, alcohol

Recently, a new treatment for peripheral neuropathy called K-Laser® is showing some promise. K-Laser® treatments are drug free, surgery free, and pain free. They use specific wavelengths of red and near-infrared light to create such therapeutic effects as: pain reduction, increased circulation, decreased swelling, and an improved healing time. Since the 1970's, K-Laser® treatments have been widely used in Europe for their healing properties by nurses and doctors. In 2002, Laser therapy was cleared for use in the United States by the FDA. It is now used here extensively.

The effectiveness of K-Laser® treatments have been demonstrated scientifically. Among its thousands of published studies, more than one hundred rigorously controlled scientific studies document the effectiveness of laser therapy for many clinical conditions, peripheral neuropathy being just one of them.

Typical treatments take only about 3 – 9 minutes each, 2 – 3 times per week, for around 5 weeks for peripheral neuropathy. Treatments for other conditions may vary from this. The treatment itself is painless with the only occasional side effect being that some old injuries may feel aggravated for a few days after treatment as the healing response becomes more active.

During therapy infrared laser light interacts with tissues on the cellular level. The metabolic activity excited within the cells effectively increases the transportation of nutrients across the cell membrane. Increased nutrients stimulate the production of cellular energy (ATP) which leads to the beneficial effects of increased cellular functioning and better health.

During each treatment laser energy draws water, oxygen, and nutrients to the affected area increasing circulation. This provides "a healing environment that reduces inflammation, swelling, muscle spasms, stiffness, and pain. As the injured area returns to normal, function is restored and pain is relieved."

References

McKay, Judith, RN, OCN. And Tamera Schacher, RN, OCN, MSN. *The Chemotherapy Survival Guide*, 3rd Edition. New harbinger Publication, Inc. Copyright © 2009 by Judith McKay and Tamera Schacher.

http://www.foodnews.org

K-Laser® brochure.

Relief from Mouth and Lip Sores

Block -- pp. 227 -- 228
"Mind-spirit techniques also reduce cancer related pain. Bone marrow transplant patients who practiced hypnosis or relaxation techniques with imagery experienced relief from severe mucositis (mouth sores) induced by chemotherapy. And focused relaxation, healing imagery, or a combination of these can dramatically improve and accelerate postsurgical repair." Pain was significantly reduced to the point where they needed less pain meds. They had fewer complications, less blood loss, quicker return to normal digestion, and shorter hospital stays.

So, where can you learn how to use these mind-body techniques?

I'm told by a psychologist friend who should absolutely know that for studying both hypnosis and relaxation techniques with guided imagery, this website is the best
Hypnosis Training College - Hypnotherapy Certification - Hypnosis Motivation Institute
(http://www.hypnosis.edu)
(This is not an affiliate link and I do not receive anything if you decide to purchase anything from them.)

Mucositis is the medical term for inflammation of the inside of your mouth. It can produce mouth sores or even ulcers that can take a long time to heal. Mouth inflammation can start forming between 5 – 10 days from your beginning therapy. It usually begins to clear up about 3 – 4 weeks after treatment ends. The time between can be difficult.

Here are some suggestions for coping:

Using toothpaste or baking soda and a child's soft toothbrush, clean your teeth and gums every morning, every evening, and after each meal.

Remove dentures and clean them every morning, every evening, and after each meal.

A warm salt water gargle might help.

Avoid mouthwashes that contain alcohol.

If you floss, be very careful not to damage your gums.

Rub a little Vaseline or lip gloss on your lips to keep them moist.

Use gravies and sauces on food to moisten it for easier swallowing.

Drink 3 pints (1 ½ liters) of fluid per day – coffee, tea, fruit & vegetable juices, soft drinks, or water.

Eating pineapple (fresh or canned) will keep your mouth fresh and moist.

Avoid acidic fruits – oranges, grapefruit, and lemons.

Chew gum

Discuss your sore mouth with your doctor. He may want to prescribe some pain killing medication.

References

Block, Keith I, M.D. *Life Over Cancer.* The Block Center Program for Integrative Cancer Treatment. Bantam Books. Copyright © 2009 by Keith I. Block, M.D. pp. 227 – 228.

http://www.hypnosis.edu

http://www.cancerresearchuk.org/about-cancer/cancers-in-general/treatment/cancer-drugs/side-effects/your-mouth-and-cancer-drugs

Relief from Dry Mouth

Sucking on ice chips was mentioned in the general help for dry mouth. Here are a few other tips that might help to keep your mouth feeling moist:

Use gravies and sauces on food to moisten it for easier swallowing.

Drink 3 pints (1 ½ liters) of fluid per day – coffee, tea, fruit & vegetable juices, soft drinks, or water.

Eating pineapple (fresh or canned) will keep your mouth fresh and moist.

Avoid acidic fruits – oranges, grapefruit, and lemons.

Chew gum

Keep a drink available and sip on it throughout the day

References

http://www.cancerresearchuk.org/about-cancer/cancers-in-general/treatment/cancer-drugs/side-effects/your-mouth-and-cancer-drugs

Protecting Nails during Chemotherapy

To reduce the possibility of nail damage during treatment, speak with your doctor before beginning chemotherapy treatments about the possibility of using cold mittens placed on the hands and feet during treatment to reduce blood flow to your nails with the hope of reducing the amount of drugs in those areas thereby reducing the likelihood of extensive damage. These have the same disadvantages as "cold caps" as discussed in the section Alopecia – Hair Loss.

Chemotherapy drugs can affect your nails. They can become dry, ridged, brittle, or develop white or dark lines on them (don't worry about the lines as they will grow out eventually). The drugs can make your nails grow slower, change your nail color, loosen them from the nail bed, or even make them fall off. Nails can flake and/or brake more easily. You can use nail oils and moisturizers. You can even use nail polish if you want to but avoid the quick-dry variety as they will dry your nails even more.

The drugs can also affect your cuticles. You may find that they fray. Don't pull at this loose skin; cut it off with clean cuticle scissors.

If you find your nails loosening from the nail bed, you must be very careful with them. Yes, they could fall off. But if they don't, they are at least providing a hospitable site for harboring bacteria. Take special care against infection by practicing excellent hygiene.

"Nail care is first line prevention for lymphedema, a condition that develops when lymph fluid accumulates in the soft tissues of the arm, causing it to swell" -- (see Relief from Fluid Retention Following Breast Surgery -- below). For those who have had underarm lymph nodes removed, pay special attention to caring for hang nails or cuts or burns on your hands or fingers as they could lead to infection and lymphedemia.

Here are a few tips for nail care during chemotherapy treatment:

Keep your nails short. Imperfections are less noticeable.

Use cuticle creams or gels instead of scissors. Don't cut your cuticles.

Massage cuticle creams onto your nails daily to help prevent hangnails, splitting and dryness.

Don't bite your nails, especially on the affected side.

Wear kitchen gloves while doing dishes. Excessive exposure to water can cause fungal infections.

For dry nails or nails that are loose or falling off, consider using daily nail moisturizer.

Use nail polish (not the fast-dry variety) to keep your nails strong and looking nice.

To remove nail polish, use a non-acetone based remover. Acetone tends to make nails dryer and dry nails are brittle and break easier.

Do not use acrylic polish.

Do not use fake nails. They trap bacteria and foster infection.

For a professional manicure, bring your own tools. You can't be too careful here.

Ask your manicurist for tips on home nail care.

Tell your doctor of any inflammation or infection.

References

http://www.cancerresearchuk.org/about-cancer/cancers-in-general/treatment/cancer-drugs/side-effects/your-skin-nails-and-cancer-drugs

http://www.breastcancer.org/tips/hair_skin_nails/nails

Relief from Fluid Retention Following Breast Cancer Surgery

Lymphedemia is the medical term which refers to fluid retention (edema) following breast surgery. The purpose of the lymphatic system in the body is to help the body's immune system fight off infections. It does this by transporting bodily fluids through its system of vessels which then filters this fluid and clears away the debris by flushing it out of the body.

Following surgery, fluid retention develops because the lymph vessels or nodes are unable to transport fluid. Perhaps they were found to be harboring metastasized cancer cells and the surgeon removed them. Or perhaps they're just clogged by too much debris and, therefore, unable to take fluid into the vessels. Either way, there is likely to be a buildup of fluids which causes swelling either in the immediate area under the armpit or in the extremities (arms and legs).

Symptoms of edema could be tightness of the skin, swelling, decreased flexibility, and/or pain. For general swelling, you may want to "ask your doctor to recommend a specially trained physical therapist who can ease the swelling and give you compression garments, exercises, and special bandages."

For edema in your feet and ankles, there are a few things that might help:

Chiropractors sometimes have vibration machines that can help get fluid flowing again. You might want to check with a chiropractor in your area about this.

Compression stockings might also help. They are available at medical supply stores and may also be purchased at drug stores.

Try to avoid cuts, burns, constriction, and muscle strain

Ask your massage therapist if she's been trained to open lymph nodes. If yes, have her gently massage your lymph nodes in the area where your upper leg connects to your body. If your lymph nodes are clogged, this might help to open them up.

For edema in your armpit:
If you still have your lymph nodes in that area, again have your specially trained massage therapist gently massage them. If they're clogged, this might help to open them up.

If the edema is painful and interfering with your arm movements, your doctor may want to physically drain the area. This could provide temporary relief.

References

http://www.webmd.com/breast-cancer/guide/side-effects-lymphedema

http://www.webmd.com/breast-cancer/advanced-bc-care-13/side-effects-tips?page=2

Conclusion

Chemotherapy side effects can be mild or devastating to the point where one wonders why someone would put themselves through all that misery. Then you look at the alternative --- and you know why.

Life. Beautiful life. Staying here a while longer. Being able to see your children grow up. Being able to grow a little older with your spouse. Yes. Beautiful life.

Hopefully, the information that has been compiled in this little booklet will help to make your journey to the other side of chemotherapy just a little better. . . . just a little easier.

Good luck . . . and see you on the other side.

Excerpt from: How to Eat Healthy

– foods to eat . . . foods to avoid

– clean eating made simple

When food is plentiful, what constitutes

CONTEMPORARY

MALNUTRITION

When a layperson hears the term 'malnutrition', we generally see in our mind's eye the picture of a person, child or adult, with rail-thin limbs, a swollen abdomen, and flies crawling all over his/her face and into the eyeballs. The person has no energy with which to raise their arm to shoo them away. However, this is only one side of malnutrition. The other is obesity. Both are deleterious. Malnutrition, therefore, can be defined as any significant nutritional deviation from that which promotes healthy bodily functioning.

Malnutrition of the body, i.e. the whole organism, begins with malnutrition of the individual cells that make up that body.

The current, traditional model for identifying malnutrition is:

Maltutrition: an insufficiency of one or more nutritional elements necessary for health and well being
-- Primary Malnutrition -- Caused by
-- (1) unavailable foodstuffs (as in poor economy, drought, or over population)

-- (2) when food is plentiful, by poor eating habits

Secondary Malnutrition -- Caused by failure of absorption of essential nutrients
i.e. – the body cannot _use_ the nutrients that are available in the foods
-- (1) as in diseases of the gastrointestinal tract, thyroid, kidney, liver, or pancreas
-- (2) by increased nutritional requirements (growth, injuries, burns, surgical procedures, pregnancy, lactation, or fever); or
-- (3) by excessive excretion (diarrhea)

This model needs to be revised to include under 'Primary Malnutrition':
-- (3) when food is plentiful **but essentially devoid of natural micro-nutrients.**

Micro-nutrients are the vitamins, minerals, phyto-chemicals, flavinoids, etc. that are present in fresh, natural, unprocessed foods. They are very delicate and are easily destroyed by heat, refining, and other processing procedures as well as by some agricultural practices.

Macro-nutrients are the fats, carbohydrates and proteins that provide the calories your body either stores as fat or uses for energy. They are very stable and not easily destroyed or altered.

When nutrition gurus talk about "nutrients", they are usually referring to the **macro-** variety – and this is where the confusion arises. Since natural food consists of BOTH micro- and macro-nutrients, and their functions in the body are very different, and you CAN eat one without the other (as in highly refined products), I think it is vitally important that professionals be very specific about which type of nutrient they're talking about.

What is the reasoning behind this proposed change?

From the beginnings of food cultivation, around 10,000 B.C., until 1840 A.D. when Liebeg introduced his NPK (nitrogen, phosphorous, potassium) theory of plant growth, the only foods (from among the hundreds of ingredients available) that were routinely consumed in the refined state (natural nutrient content either severely reduced or eliminated) were: refined sugar (dating from prior to 510 B.C.), refined white wheat flour (dating from prior to 150 B.C.), and refined olive oils, another ancient practice. The production of olive oil began around 5,000 B.C., but I have not yet found a definitive date for when it began to be widely used as a refined product. These were, and are, staple foods.

When these were the primary natural micro-nutrient deficient foods consumed on a regular basis, the impact to the nutrition of the cells was low. (Food preservation, another ancient practice, also somewhat reduced natural micro-nutrient content but not nearly as severely as refining.) The ingestion of a greater majority of untreated, micro-nutrient-rich foods has the effect of "making up for" the nutrient deficiencies of the treated foods.

It is postulated that sugars entering the cells that do not contain sufficient natural micro-nutrients to adequately . . .

#

End of Excerpt. *How to Eat Healthy – foods to eat . . . foods to avoid* – clean eating made simple
is available at Amazon.com. Click the link to be taken to its page. You can continue reading in just a few seconds.

DISCLAIMER

The information in this booklet is for informational purposes only. The author is NOT a medical professional and none of the information here is intended to diagnose or treat any condition or take the place of the council and advice of

This book is presented solely for informational and educational purposes so you can learn more about the subject.

The information provided in *Chemotherapy Relief* is NOT INTENDED TO PROVIDE MEDICAL ADVICE OR TREAT OR CURE ANY DISEASE OR HEALTH PROBLEM OR OFFER ANY SPECIFIC DIAGNOSIS TO ANY INDIVIDUAL. You should always consult your licensed healthcare professional before making significant changes to your diet or taking any form of medication.

I am NOT a licensed healthcare professional. My background and degrees are in Clinical Psychology and Certified Professional Coaching. However, I have had college level training in biology, human physiology and nutrition and have done extensive independent research in nutrition.

While I have made significant effort to provide accurate information, the information provided here should NOT be considered complete and exhaustive of the topic and I DISCLAIM ANY LIABILITY OR LOSS IN CONNECTION WITH YOUR USE OF THE INFORMATION CONTAINED HEREIN. YOUR USE OF ANY INFORMATION PROVIDED HERE IS TOTALLY YOUR RESPONSIBILITY.

You should never disregard medical advice or delay in seeking it because of something you have read here. This information is not intended as and should not be used in place of a visit to or consultation with or the advice of a physician or other qualified health care provider.

About the Author

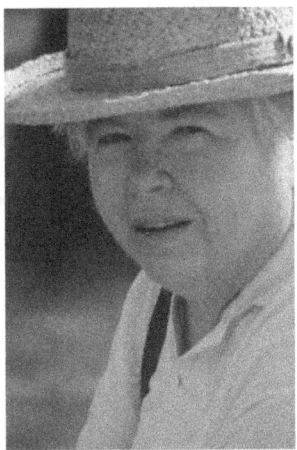

In 1975, my husband, two little baby girls, and I were living in an apartment in Chicago's Hyde Park district. My husband had diabetes and asthma and I realized I didn't know very much about healthy food and the best way to feed my family. I'd always been a fairly decent student having graduated a few years earlier with a M.A. degree from Bradley University in clinical psychology.

I minored in biology as an undergraduate and did postgraduate work in biology with an emphasis on human anatomy and physiology. I've also done considerable independent study in this area as well as studying about foods simply because I enjoy it and to help my husband with his Type 2 Diabetes. My latest book, *How to Eat Healthy – foods to eat . . . foods to avoid* is available at on Amazon.

One Last Thing Before You Go..
.

Thank you for purchasing **Chemotherapy Relief** – *Research results to protect you from chemo side effects.* If you enjoyed it or found it useful, would you take a few moments and write a short review on its Amazon page?

If you believe the book is worth sharing, also let your friends know about it on Twitter and Facebook? If it turns out to make a difference in their lives, they'll be forever grateful to you.

As will I.

All the best
Joyce Zborower

Amazon Top 3 Bestsellers in Cancer

(October 24, 2014)

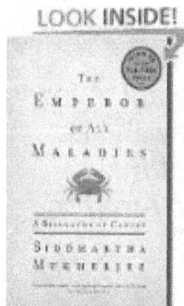

The Emperor of All Maladies: A Biogra...
by Siddhartha Mukherjee

4.7 out of 5 stars **(923)**
Kindle Edition

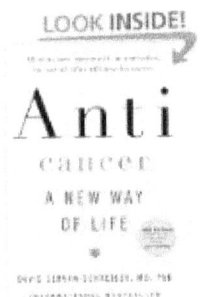

Anticancer, A New Way of Life, New Ed...
by David Servan-Schreiber MD PhD
4.8 out of 5 stars **(440)**
Kindle Edition

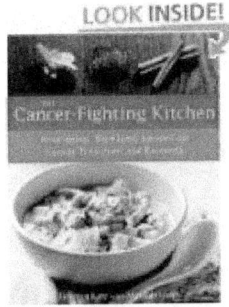

The Cancer-Fighting Kitchen: Nourishi...
by Rebecca Katz
4.6 out of 5 stars **(280)**
Kindle Edition

Recommended Books

--AUDIO-BOOKS

The Truth about Olive Oil – Benefits, Curing Methods, Remedies
Signs of Vitamin B12 Deficiencies – Who's at Risk – Why – What Can Be Done
No Work Urban Front Yard Vegetable Gardening Simplified – for in-ground, raised or container gardening
Homebrew Beer – Experience tantalizing tastes from unique beer making ingredients by Eric Andrews
Sell Your Work – Report: How to Turn Your Craft into Your Business
How to Fight Depression – 9 Case Studies by John F. Walsh, M.S. and Joyce Zborower, M.A.
My Cushings Journey – A True Story by Karen Rhodes
Chemotherapy Relief – Chemotherapy research to protect you from chemo side effects
Basic Ab Workouts Give You Sexy Flat Abs – Your one stop flat abs resource – by Michael Weston

--AUDIO-BOOK GAME GUIDES

Piano Tiles Game: Cheats, Online, Mod, Apk, Download Guide – HiddenStuff Entertainment
Subway Surfers: Tips, Cheats, Tricks, & Strategies – HiddenStuff Entertainment
8 Ball Pool Game: How to Download for Android, PC, IOS, Kindle + Tips – HiddenStuff Entertainment
The Sims Free Play Game Guide – HiddenStuff Entertainment

--FOOD AND NUTRITION RELATED BOOKS

Paleo Slow Cooker Cookbook – 31 low carb and/or gluten free paleo slow cooker recipes for busy folks who love homemade food by Julie A. Anderson

25 Crockpot Meals with MEAT –Delicious, easy, healthy Crockpot Meals with Meat (beef and pork) in 3 Steps or Less by Julie A. Anderson

25 Crockpot Meals with CHICKEN – Delicious, easy, healthy Crockpot Chicken Recipes in 3 Steps or Less by Julie A. Anderson

25 Crockpot Meals for BREAKFAST – Delicious, easy, healthy Crockpot Breakfast Recipes in 3 Steps or Less by Julie A. Anderson

75 Crockpot Meals Cookbook in 3 Steps or Less by Julie A. Anderson – 3 book set

Meat – Chicken -- Breakfast

Delicious Dinner and Dessert Pie – Pie recipes for quick and easy pies and pie crust -- by Julie A. Anderson

Homebrew Beer – How to brew beer right the first time and experience tantalizing tastes from unique beer making ingredients -- by Eric Andrews

No Work Vegetable Gardening – for in-ground, raised, or container gardening

3 Fruit Pie Recipes – apple, cherry, crisp persimmon

How to Eat Healthy – foods to eat . . . foods to avoid – clean eating made simple

The Truth About Olive Oil – benefits, curing methods, remedies

External Uses of Extra Virgin Olive Oil – Folk Remedies ... Body Lotions ... Pet Treatments

Signs of Vitamin B12 Deficiencies – Who's at Risk – Why – What Can Be Done

13 Easy Tomato Recipes – nature's lycopene rich superfood for heart health and cancer protection

BBQ Spare Ribs Recipe – with homemade honey BBQ sauce

-- HEALTH & FITNESS/EXERCISE BOOKS – by

Michael Weston

Basic Ab Workouts Give You Sexy Flat Abs --- by Michael Weston

Ab Workouts For Skinny Guys Who Want To Build Some Muscle and Turn Some Heads Even If You've Never Been Able To Do That With Other Workout Programs ---- by Michael Weston

-- MYSTERIES/SHORT STORIES

Mango Muffin Murder – Island Kitchen Cozy Culinary Mystery by Emma Johns – Book1 Jamaica Series

Murder by Mistake -- Island Kitchen Cozy Culinary Mystery by Emma Johns – Book2 Jamaica Series

The Trust – a cautionary tale

Little Mysteries – a short story

-- CRAFTS BOOKS – by Joyce Zborower

Handcrafted Jewelry Step by Step – 6 advanced and intermediate original designs

Handcrafted Jewelry Photo Gallery – cast jewelry -- fabricated jewelry

Wire Jewelry Photo Gallery – Original designs

Creations in Wood Photo Gallery – jewelry boxes, screens, storage ideas

Bargello Quilts Photo Gallery – quilt wall hangings

Bargello Train Quilt – cutting and sewing instructions

Sell Your Work – how to turn your craft into your business

-- SELF-HELP BOOKS – by Joyce

Zborower and/or John F. Walsh

Chemotherapy Relief – Chemotherapy research results to protect you from chemo side effects

Psychology of Success – RESEARCH -- How to have success when trying to change how you look

Different Types of Depression – Characteristics and Treatments by Joyce Zborower and John F. Walsh

How to Fight Depression – 9 case studies ---- by John F. Walsh

Clinical Psychology – A Professional Perspective – memoirs and experiences – John F. Walsh

-- CHILDREN'S BOOKS – by Joyce Zborower

Baby Pics Counting and Number Book -- 1-13 The numbers are in numerals and words with lots of photos of babies.

Christmas ABCs – cute animal illustrations

Most of the above are also available as print-on-demand paperback editions. Also:

Grandma's No Work Vegetable Gardening – (paperback edition) same as *No Work Vegetable Gardening* except the photos are B&W and the price is lower.

-- Español Libros (Spanish language Books)

-- by Joyce Zborower and M. Angelica Brunell S.

Haga click aquí para ir a mi página de Amazon

Pequeños Misterios – cuento

Joyas Artesanales Galeria de fotos – Joyas fundidas – joyas forjadas

Joyas de Alambre - Galería de fotos – Diseños originales

Creaciones en Madera- Galería de fotos – joyeros, biombos, ideas de almacenaje

Quilts Estilo Bargello - Galería de fotos – tapices de quilt

Bargello **Quilt de Tren** – instrucciones para cortar y coser
Vende tuTrabajo – como transformar tu arte en negocio
Signos de deficiencia de vitamina B12 -- Quén esta en riesgo – Por qué – Qué puede hacerse
Huerto sin Esfuerzo – para jardinería en el suelo, elevada o en contenedor
La Verdad Acerca del Aceite de Oliva – beneficios, métodos de curación, remedios
3 Recetas de Pie de Fruta -- Manzana, Cereza, Caqui fresco
13 Recetas de Tomate Fáciles -- Superalimentos de la naturaleza ricos en licopeno para la salud del corazón y protección contra el cáncer
Receta de Chuletas de Cerdo en Barbacoa -- con salsa casera de barbacoa con miel
Fotos de Bebés Libro de Números y de Contar De 2 a 5 años – 1 – 13
ABCs de Navidad – Para niños de 2 a 5 años

-- Other Recommended Books

Romance Books by Nicole Ann Drake

**** WARNING ****

These books by Nicole Ann Drake contain sexually explicit scenes and adult language. They may be considered offensive to some readers. These books are for sale to adults ONLY.
(Must be 18 or older.)

Sexy Romance Novellas
.....**Teacher's Pet** – a love story
   Boardroom Beauty – a love story
Wedding Party Series – Sexy Romance Short Stories
All the characters in the series connect at wedding related events with the event from the previous story forming the base for the next story.
   Wedding Party Series (Compilation Books 1 thru 6)
   Once Burnt – Twice Shy (Book 1 – Wedding Party Series)
   Just One Night (Book 2 – Wedding Party Series)

The Event Planner's Event (Book 3 – Wedding Party Series)

The Playboy's Physician (Book 4 – Wedding Party Series)

Heart Song (Book 5 – Wedding Party Series)

Pleasures Postponed (Book 6 – Wedding Party Series)

Tammy the Tabby Series – Hot Romance Short Stories

There is a stray cat in the neighborhood that everyone nicknames 'Tammy'. Every now and then she attaches herself to a particular household. The persons to whom she attaches herself have their love story told. When their issues are resolved she moves on to someone else.

Tammy the Tabby -- Book (Compilation Books 1 thru 6)

Keeper of the Books (Book 1 – Tammy the Tabby Series)

Doctor's Orders (Book 2 – Tammy the Tabby Series)

This Little Piggy (Book 3 – Tammy the Tabby Series)

Moving On (Book 4 – Tammy the Tabby Series)

Better Late than Never (Book 5 – Tammy the Tabby Series)

Full Circle (Book 6 – Tammy the Tabby Series)

The Confession of a Trust Magnate ----- by George Allen Yuille

Picture the combined navies of the world
anchored off our seaboard cities, the
combined armies of the world in possession
of our inland cities, envoys from each
nation congregated at Washington
partitioning our country, the entire population
being apportioned as slaves to do the bidding
of the conquerors.
Would you be interested?
An equally appalling situation confronts
the people of this country to-day.
Read of it in the pages of this book.

This book by George Allen Yuille was written in 1911. Its message is critical for today – 2014.

#

If you enjoyed this book, please leave a review on its Amazon page.

For Chemo Turban Hats
And other Chemotherapy Patient Supplies
Visit

http://headgearexpress.com

.

www.ingramcontent.com/pod-product-compliance
Lightning Source LLC
Chambersburg PA
CBHW070411190526
45169CB00003B/1212